Pregnancy the Green Family Way

How to Have a Baby While Still Being Earth-Friendly

Teagan Smith

equally by a Committee of the American Bar Association and a Committee of Publishers and Associations.

The information provided herein is stated to be truthful and consistent, in that any liability, in terms of inattention or otherwise,

Contents

Chapter 1 - What are the common symptoms of pregnancy?

First we are going to focus on what the most common symptoms of pregnancy are.

1.   Breasts: One of the most important symptoms for pregnancy is the changing of breasts. If anyone is going to be pregnant, her breasts may be swollen, tender or tingling.

2.   Nausea: Morning sickness is quite common and can happen at different times throughout the day. Usually this caused by an increase in hormones but can also be linked to things such as smells of certain foods,

tea, coffee, smoke and other things. This is usually a common indicator of being pregnant.

3. Breathing: You may experience short breathing, which is also another common symptom to pregnancy. As your baby starts to grow, your lungs may not be able to expand as much as they usually do. This usually is experienced in the second trimester.

4. Fatigue: The increase of hormones will cause most during pregnancy to feel

extremely tired. This is normal and should be expected.

5. Urinating frequently: Extra fluids are being produced by your body when you are pregnant. Your body needs to work more when you are pregnant so your body will produce urine more frequently.

6. Headaches and backaches: Another common symptom of pregnancy is headaches or backaches. Due to the increasing of hormones, these headaches occur and are due to the loosening of ligaments.

Chapter 2 – Best practices

You will want to follow some best practices once you find out that you are pregnant.

1. Alert your companion: Your first duty is to send the news of your pregnancy to your life partner, as they will help you greatly during this time. During this time you will want to have as much help as you can.

2. Get enough sleep: It is important to get at least 8 to 10 hours of sleep every night. This is crucial for yourself as you are

carrying the baby and for the baby's development as well.

3.   Have necessary foods: Foods play a great role in the case of having a good pregnancy. Make sure you are eating right on a daily basis. Junk foods and fast foods are not recommended. Eat healthy foods like fruits, fishes, and vegetables, which are essential for the health of you and your baby as well. It is important to eat foods that contain protein, which can be found in food such as eggs, peanuts, beans, and meat. Protein plays an important role

in that it helps to increase the ability for the growth of cells and for the production of blood as well.

4.   Have calcium: Another important matter is that you have to have enough calcium at the time of pregnancy. The development of nerve, fetus and bone is highly dependent on calcium. Calcium can be found in foods such as spinach, milk, yogurt and hard cheeses. It is mandatory for you to get a minimum of 1000 mg calcium daily during pregnancy.

5. Make changes in what you wear: Wear clothes which are comfortable to wear and not overly tight. You need to wear soft, looser clothes such as blouses that will allow for plenty of room.

6. Practice exercises: Make a schedule to exercise, which will keep you even healthier. Consult with a physician to help figure out what will be the best exercise types to take part in during this time.

7. Take time out in the day for yourself: You will have to rest for long periods in each day.

This can be done by sleeping, exercising and relaxing. You can also do things such as yoga, deep breathing, visualization, massage and meditation.

8.   Make a schedule: Make a schedule so that it is easy to remember all the required things that must be done when you are pregnant. Include times for eating, taking rest, sleeping and other activities in your schedule.

Chapter 3 – Tips and Tricks

Here are some helpful things to know for your pregnancy.

1. Get iron naturally: Although you can get iron from medical supplements prescribed by a doctor, it is better for you to get it from natural sources. Iron helps with blood cell production. You can also get iron from cereals, breads, spinach, and meat.

2. Don't feel shy: Tell others about your pregnancy so that they can help you.

3. Be toxin free: Today various types of natural remedies are available to help become toxin free. If you can start eating healthy foods, it will help to reduce toxins from your body.

4. Avoid using nail polishes: You will want to give up the habit of using nail polishes in order to have a green pregnancy. Nail polish can contain many toxins such as toluene and formaldehyde.

5.   Avoid plastics: Avoid the habit of using plastics to store water or other supplements. Plastic contains some toxins like BPA, which is harmful for both you and your baby.

Chapter 4 – Meals for a green pregnancy

Here are some ideas of food you could eat to stay healthy during your pregnancy.

1. Fish: Fish can be a helpful food when you are pregnant. It can be a fabulous source of protein and DHA as well. It is best to stick to types of fish such as cod, flounder, and wild salmon.

2. Veggie omelet: Veggie omelets are a great way to spice up breakfast in a healthy way. You can use vegetables such as

onions, spinach and tomatoes. Feel free to use herbs like oregano, basil and chives that will increase the flavor of your omelet.

3. Veggie Pizza: You can also add veggie pizza in your daily meal plan to have a more enjoyable pregnancy. You can make the pizza by baking in tomatoes, spinach, basil, cubed chicken and red peppers. Parmesan and skim mozzarella can be used as additional ingredients.

Remember that your appetite will be greater than any other time in your life so far. It is important to be focused on eating healthy for the sake of yourself during the delivery and for your baby's health as well.

Chapter 5 – Bad habits to avoid

There are many things that you will not want to do once you realize that you are pregnant. This is for the benefit of your unborn child. Your sacrifice will be rewarded once you see the smile of your healthy newborn child.

1.   Smoking: Smoking can easily damage your lungs but also the lungs of your baby as well. It is highly important to not have this be part of your pregnancy.

2. Alcohol: Please do not drink during your pregnancy, as the effects of alcohol on an unborn child are catastrophic. The child can be prone to Fetal Alcohol Spectrum Disorders, which can include things such as brain damage and birth defects.

3. Drugs: Partaking in illegal drugs such as cocaine and heroin can cause debilitating effects to an unborn child. They can range from brain bleeding to sudden infant death syndrome.

4. Caffeine: Many of our favorite drinks like coffee, tea

and soda contain caffeine, which is harmful for you at the time of pregnancy. Caffeine consumption can cause issues in newborns such as bone loss and sudden infant death syndrome.

Do what is best for your unborn child by taking up a different lifestyle as soon as you find out you are pregnant. It will be better for your family in the long run, I guarantee it!

Conclusion

Thank you for reading this book. My hope is that it gives you a starting point in your journey to having a successful green pregnancy.

Your little one will thank you for it one day, you can be sure of that!